Contents

PRESENTATION 4
SECTION ONE 6
What is the Mayr Method Diet? 6
The Mayr Method Explained 7
   The Mayr Method Foods and Nutrition 7
      Mayr Method Breakfast 9
      Mindful Eating and Awareness 9
      Mayr Method Chewing 10
   Can I Lose Weight with the Mayr Method Diet? 11
   How the Mayr Method Works 12
   Possible Advantages of the Mayr Method 13
   Disadvantages of the Mayr Method 15
   Should You Try the Mayr Method for Weight Loss? 17
SECTION TWO 19
How to Start the Mayr Method if Your Doctor Okays It
.... 19
   What is the Mayr Method Diet and Is It Right for You?
   20
   What is the Mayr Method Diet? 21
   What Should I Expect When Following the Mayr
   Method Diet? 22
   Is the Mayr Method Diet Safe and Effective? 25
   Are There Better Ways to Get Similar Benefits? 29

- Is the Mayr Method Diet Right for You? 36
- What's the Best Gut Health Diet? 37
- CHAPTER THREE 52
- Intermittent Fasting 52
- What is intermittent fasting and does it actually work? 52
- What is intermittent fasting? 52
  - Does it work for weight loss? 54
    - Other benefits 56
    - Potential downsides 57
  - How Intermittent Fasting Can Help You Lose Weight 59
    - The 16/8 method 60
    - The 5:2 method 62
    - Eat Stop Eat 64
    - Alternate-day fasting 65
    - The Warrior diets 67
- The Takeaway: Is the Mayr Method Healthy? 68
- CONCLUSION 70

Copyright ©2021. WILFRED DAWSON

All rights reserved. No part of this publication may be reproduced, distributed, or transmitted in any form or by any means, including photocopying, recording, or other electronic or mechanical methods, without the prior written permission of the publisher, except in the case of brief quotations embodied in critical reviews and certain other noncommercial uses permitted by copyright law.

PRESENTATION

After declaring 2020 her "Year of Health" and sharing a weight loss goal earlier in the year, Rebel Wilson has given her Instagram adherents an inside look into her new diet and wellness routine. The Pitch Perfect star had beforehand said she needed to hit 75 kilograms, about 165 pounds, by the end of the year. Recently, Rebel delighted her fans when she revealed that she had achieved her objective a month ahead of schedule.

Having spent her Thanksgiving occasion at the notable wellness focus VivaMayr, the 40-year-old actress as of late shared a snapshot of her scale on location in Austria by means of her Instagram Story.

"Hit my goal with one month to spare!" she posted, adding, "Even however it's not about a weight number, it's about being solid, I needed a tangible measurement to have as a goal and that was 75 kg.

The Mayr strategy attracted consideration after the actor Rebel Wilson credited it with her late weight misfortune. To follow this eating plan, you'll need to sign up for a stay at one of the VivaMayr luxury resorts, where mentors will prescribe you a "cure" based on four columns: medication, nourishment, work out, and mindfulness. This holistic approach to weight loss may combine treatments such as oxygen therapy, nourishing discussion, water cycling, and personal training, per their website, however the individual medicines will change depending on your decision of plan.

That being stated, this is not a doable weight misfortune plan for most people, mainly because you will need to travel to a Mayr clinic to receive treatment — which can be expensive, tedious, and subject to travel restrictions during the COVID-19 pandemic. Moreover, while you're likely to make progress on such an vivid retreat, it may be difficult to sustain your weight loss once the retreat has finished and you return to your typical daily practice. Last however not least, numerous of the revealed therapies used on these withdraws, including laxatives, are not a safe way to get more fit, some experts warn.

SECTION ONE

What is the Mayr Method Diet?

The Mayr Method was made almost 100 years ago by Dr. Franz Xaver Mayr, an Austrian doctor.

Mayr created the program based on the conviction that people damage their digestive systems with what they eat and how they eat. So, by cleaning up your act as far as gut health, you can be healthier and lose weight.

Dr. Mayr believed that by changing our normal diet and practicing fasting routinely, we can achieve more noteworthy wellbeing.

For a program that's been around nearly 100 years, I was astounded that I'd never heard of it.

The Mayr Method Explained

The Mayr Diet centers on what you eat and how you eat it. The basic precepts of this program include eating an soluble diet, dispensing with specific nourishments, expanding your care around mealtimes, and chewing your food thoroughly.

The Mayr Method Foods and Nutrition

This aspect of the program focuses on great gut health. In the event that you've been around here for some time, you know that gut wellbeing is SO important to overall health. A good gut health diet is the foundation of living a solid, dynamic life.

While some of the things outlined in this diet may seem prohibitive, many do make sense from a gut wellbeing standpoint.

• Eliminating sugar, caffeine, and alcohol: Sugar, caffeine, and liquor are no-noes for this program, so the Mayr strategy commences by eliminating these offenders. Considering a sugar and/or caffeine detox isn't an impractical notion, particularly if you are eating a huge load of simple sugars and are continually having to have a mug of espresso to get through your evening.

• Eating an eating routine composed of entire foods that are highly alkaline. A basic diet is one that includes basic foods like broccoli and acidic ones like lemons that advance alkalinity in your body.

• Eliminating dairy and gluten.

• Eliminating snacking throughout the day which lets your digestive framework rest between meals.

• Eating breakfast. Which implies dispensing with supper if you're intermittent fasting.

- No raw foods following 4 pm around evening time.

- No drinking with suppers. Burn-through all beverages between dinners.

Mayr Method Breakfast

This strategy encourages you to eat your largest dinner at breakfast, a smaller meal at lunch and an even smaller meal at dinner. So if you're a breakfast lover, this program may be worth a try for you.

On the off chance that you are incorporating discontinuous fasting into your plan, you will need to switch your schedule so you eat breakfast and skip dinner.

Mindful Eating and Awareness

A important part of the Mayr method involves improving your awareness of food, being careful while eating, and thoroughly biting each nibble. You'll need to stick to these guidelines if you need to follow the Mayr diet method:

• Never eat on the go. Stop, sit down and relish each bite.

• Eat slowly.

• Stop eating when you feel full.

• Eliminate distractions while eating. This implies no TV, no cell phone, no reading. Nothing to distract you from being fully present and careful during dinners.

Mayr Method Chewing

One especially extraordinary perspective of this program involves chewing each bite of food at least 40 times. Not only does chewing start the digestive process, however it has been considered and shown to help you eat less calories.

Since you shouldn't be distracted with anything during meals, you'll be ready to center on spending your time counting each and each bite.

Can I Lose Weight with the Mayr Method Diet?

On the off chance that you have a few thousand dollars to spend (not including airfare or inn!), you may need to look at the luxury Austrian resort/spa called the "Viva Mayr" that caters to the rich and famous who want to lose weight and improve their health.

Fortunately, if you're interested in the Mayr diet, you don't have to spend big bucks at an European health spa. The Vaya Mayr resort published a book you can get on Amazon that plots the measure and promises "14 days to a compliment stomach and a younger you!"

How the Mayr Method Works

You can sign up for the Mayr method by booking a stay at one of the VivaMayr luxury "medi-clinics" and resorts. The Mayr method is a plan that treats your body and mind as a whole. According to the Original FX Mayr website, which refers to it as the "FX Mayr cure," the program is "based on four pillars: medicine, nourishment, exercise, and awareness." Treatments for their wellness programs might incorporate a clinical assessment, metabolic and urine examination, given food, detoxing, body wraps, knead, dietary advice, a colonoscopy, and more. For people looking to lose weight, there is a specific weight loss program, which incorporates both unproven treatments like oxygen therapy and "fat burning infusions" as well as customary weight misfortune direction like nutrition consultation and personal training.

The details on precisely what is done in the eating regimen are a bit murky; this is a program offered at an expensive medical clinic and spa. That doesn't mean you can't receive the principles and lessons and apply them to your own life no matter where you are, however there isn't a strict blueprint or set of guidelines for how to do so.

Possible Advantages of the Mayr Method

The food that's provided is based on "fresh, seasonal, and provincial ingredients," according to the Original FX Mayr. A plant-put together diet centered with respect to supplement rich foods such as vegetables is certainly health promoting, says Emmaline Rasmussen, RDN, the owner of Sound Nutrition in Chicago. Individuals who follow a plant-based diet have a 19 and 11 percent lower hazard, respectively, of death from cardiovascular disease and any other cause, as compared with individuals who eat fewer plants and more creature items, according to an investigation published August 2019 in the Journal of the American Heart Association.

Mayr also advances mindful eating. Harvard Women's Health Watch characterizes this as eating without interruptions, stopping to value your food before you eat it, taking small bites, and gradually (and completely) chewing to savor the aromas and surfaces of your food. According to People.com, resortgoers are instructed to chew their food 30 times before swallowing. "Careful eating is a game changer, [when] you delayed down and remove external improvements, as the TV or telephone from the dinner table. When your eyes are not looking at your food, you're not intellectually enrolling what's on your plate," Rasmussen clarifies. In a little randomized controlled preliminary published in the Journal of Family Medicine and Community Health in June 2018, adults who finished a 15-week get-healthy plan, which included training in mindfulness eating, lost about four pounds looked at with a control bunch that lost about a half pound.

That said, 30 times is a ton. It would likely be tiring and likewise would turn your food into fluid, thus destroying its surface and flavor, which is among life's pleasures. "This rule feels a little fanatical and rings of scattered eating," says Rasmussen.

Last, there is an accentuation on both pressure and sleep, as part of the whole-body approach. That is a tremendous positive. Research published in the International Journal of Obesity in June 2019 on almost 2,000 adults found that over the course of a year, people who stalled out to a more consistent schedule were more successful in losing weight. As for stress, a small study distributed in the Journal of Molecular Biochemistry in December 2018 concluded that adults at a medical obesity clinic who attended an eight-week stress management program (focused on deep breathing, progressive muscle relaxation, and guided visualization) decreased their BMI more than the control group, and reduced despondency and uneasiness for sure.

Disadvantages of the Mayr Method

One of the bigger problems with Mayr is that you're supposed to travel to one of the medical clinics that offer the Mayr method and stay there for some time. That has its own limitations in terms of expense, resources (including time), and the current COVID-19 pandemic, which has created travel concerns and restrictions. It is tempting to think that if you could just go somewhere for a week or two, you might come out of it with your diet and lifestyle habits permanently transformed.

Mayr is one of many strict diets without proven results. "These quick-fix ideas are appealing. People are feeling discouraged with their current situation, and having a set of rules or restrictions imposed on you sounds really desirable," says the New York City–based nutrition and wellness expert Samantha Cassetty, RD, the coauthor of Sugar Shock.

What's more, other treatments touted by Mayr, including cryotherapy and massage, are unproven to help you lose weight or release toxins, says Rasmussen. And the method as a whole does not have any research behind it, which is another downside.

The Toronto-based registered dietitian Abby Langer writes on her blog that you may even experience serious illness from some of the reported tenets of Mayr, which include bloodletting, severe calorie restriction (600 calories a day), and laxatives.

Beyond these potentially dangerous therapies, a trip to any sort of wellness retreat that touts weight loss as an end goal is not likely to provide sustainable results, says Rasmussen. "When you get back to regular life, everyday stresses and being surrounded by fast food, snacks, and processed food will make it really tough to maintain any weight loss. If this center is not just removing stimuli and temptations and is teaching long-term healthy behaviors that you can apply to your life outside, then you may be successful," she says. Put differently, in real life, you won't have a chef make meals for you, a resort that controls everything you eat, and massages at the ready, so it's unlikely that you'll be able to maintain that brand-new you.

Should You Try the Mayr Method for Weight Loss?

You don't need to try the Mayr method, says Cassetty. While it may be worth adopting some of the positive elements of the program, like slowing down your eating and eating mindfully, you can do without most of it.

In the beginning of the diet, you'll be required to fast, cleanse, restrict the foods you're eating, and take vitamin and mineral supplements, according to Today.com. This is a huge red flag. Not only do you have working organs that do these jobs, but detoxing hasn't been shown to be a viable long-term strategy for good health or weight loss. "If we look at the people who live the longest, healthiest lives in the world, they are not doing detoxes. They adhere to healthy pillars of a plant-focused diet that includes pulses and vegetables, limit their alcohol, get movement in their daily life, and nourish their social connections and sense of community," says Cassetty. "When we look at the whole picture, we know people do not need to detox to be healthy."

SECTION TWO

How to Start the Mayr Method if Your Doctor Okays It

It's not feasible for a large portion of us to pack up and attend a expensive wellness program at a medical spa in Austria. (What might be compared to about $1,800 for a seven-day stay.

Instead, as long as your medical care team Okays it, you can start with the book The Viva Mayr Diet: 14 Days to a Flatter Stomach and a Younger You. The book was written by Harald Stossier, who is the head of the VivaMayr Maria Wörth medi-clinic in Austria and is considered to be the mind behind the program, and it was published in 2010. The book includes guidelines for following the diet. For model, in case you're choosing between wine and water at dinner, drink wine each time, eat more carefully and with goal, and eat breakfast yet make supper optional. This advice appears to be a bit different from what you'd receive at one of the wellness retreats, as alcohol is not permitted during the program. However, the book appears to be a attempt to bring the plan more into the real world and make it more doable.

What is the Mayr Method Diet and Is It Right for You?

If you're trying to drop weight, you may have heard about the Mayr Method diet but are wondering if this type of weight loss plan is safe and effective.

There are A LOT of fad diets and it can be hard to tell what's real or what's just a gimmick.

We've discovered the proven path to help you lose weight and get healthy while balancing your busy life and helping your family live healthier too.

Still, there's a lot of information (and misinformation) out there, so we want to try and help educate you on everything.

Knowing more about the Mayr Method diet and if it's right for you can help you meet health, fitness, and weight loss goals!

Here's what you need to know.

What is the Mayr Method Diet?

The Mayr Method diet plan, also known as Viva Mayr Diet, is based on the Mayr Cure, which was created by Austrian physician Franz Xaver Mayr, MD, 100 years ago.

Some celebrities, including Rebel Wilson, have effectively lost weight while following the Mayr Method plan.

This type of weight loss diet includes four key components:

• Nutrition and gut health

• Exercise

• Medicine

• Awareness

It's based on the belief that people poison their digestive systems with typical eating patterns and foods.

The Mayr Method plan combines traditional therapies with complementary medicine to treat health problems, if they exist, and use exercise plus proper nutrition to improve mental awareness.

Mayr Method diet creators tout a flatter stomach, more energy, and glowing skin.

What Should I Expect When Following the Mayr Method Diet?

When following the Mayr Method diet for weight loss, you focus on improving gut and overall health and wellness.

Plan to make the following changes when following Mayr Method eating plans:

Nutrition and Gut Health

Use the following nutritional guidelines when following the Mayr Method for weight loss:

• Begin the program with sugar and caffeine detox

• Stop snacking

• Reduce your intake of dairy foods

- Reduce your consumption of gluten-containing foods, including wheat, barley, and rye food products

- Chew foods for a longer period of time (chew each bite of food 40-60 times)

- Eat high-alkaline whole foods like fruits, vegetables, tofu, nuts, seeds, legumes, and fish

- Avoid highly processed foods

- Focus on mindfulness while eating

The bottom line is you'll eat mainly healthy, whole foods when following the Mayr Method diet and eat fewer calories overall.

Exercise

There's more to the Mayr Method weight loss plan than simply changing up your dietary habits.

You'll exercise regularly, up to six days per week, in addition to eating healthy foods.

Combine cardiovascular workouts with resistance training to achieve optimal results.

Medicine

Getting the right medical treatment for chronic disease risk factors can significantly reduce your chance of developing a debilitating condition, such as diabetes, heart disease, or cancer.

See your doctor regularly to properly control your blood pressure, cholesterol, or triglycerides with medical treatment when necessary in addition to making healthy lifestyle changes.

If your doctor recommends you take medicines for chronic diseases, you may be able to reduce your dosage or eliminate the need for medications altogether as you begin losing weight.

Awareness

Each time you eat food, focus on the task at hand to avoid being distracted and eating too many calories overall.

Common distractions can include playing with your phone, watching television, reading, and talking on the phone or with friends.

Is the Mayr Method Diet Safe and Effective?

As long as you don't severely restrict calories or foods when following the Mayr Method diet, this way of eating can be safe and effective.

Here are the keys to the diet:

Eat Alkaline Foods

Many whole, minimally processed foods like fruits, vegetables, legumes, and nuts, are naturally more alkaline, which is why eating alkaline foods when choosing the Mayr Method diet is a good idea.

However, you don't have to only eat alkaline foods because if you're in good health, your body can properly manage pH levels on its own.

Chew Each Bite of Food 40-60 Times

Chewing each bite of food 40-60 times is tedious and time-consuming, and not realistic in every situation.

However, this strategy might help you eat slower and consume fewer calories overall, which is beneficial when you're trying to achieve your goal weight.

Nix Sugar and Caffeine

Eliminating sugar is an excellent healthy eating strategy, but reducing caffeine when you're used to drinking coffee or tea can drain your energy.

In fact, studies show that caffeine can increase your metabolism, aid in weight loss, and reduce body mass index (BMI) and body fat.

Avoid caffeinated sodas, however, as they contain added sugar that can contribute to unwanted weight gain.

Avoid Snacks

Avoiding snacks is one way to reduce your overall calorie intake for weight loss, as long as you don't overindulge at mealtime.

However, you don't have to skip snacks entirely to effectively drop weight.

In fact, not eating snacks can lead to between-meal fatigue or overindulging at mealtime in some instances.

Eat a small meal or snack every few hours or so.

Reduce Dairy Foods

Reducing your intake of dairy foods, as recommended by creators of the Mayr Method diet plan, isn't necessary to shed excess weight.

In fact, low-fat dairy foods like Greek yogurt, low-fat cottage cheese, and low-fat milk offer you high-quality protein, calcium, and vitamin D your body needs to function properly.

Studies show that eating calcium-rich dairy foods appears to enhance weight loss and improve body composition in women trying to lose weight.

So, nixing dairy foods isn't necessary but if you prefer to avoid them, choose calcium-fortified plant milks or yogurts instead.

Avoid Gluten

Avoiding foods with gluten isn't necessary for weight loss either, though you should avoid wheat, barley, and rye products if you have Celiac disease or gluten sensitivity.

Steer clear of highly processed gluten-containing products, however, such as white bread.

Practice Mindfulness

Using mindfulness, as recommended by creators of the Mayr Method diet, is often an effective weight loss solution.

While you don't have to chew your food a certain number of times to consume fewer calories, eating slowly is a good weight loss strategy.

So is not being distracted while eating.

Are There Better Ways to Get Similar Benefits?

If the Mayr Method diet seems too restrictive and you'd prefer a meal plan you can stick with long-term.

When following this type of well-balanced, healthy lifestyle plan for weight loss, expect to:

Eat a Variety of Healthy Foods

The Fit Mother Project plan is well-balanced, meaning you'll eat a wide variety of nutritious foods like:

- Fruits
- Non-starchy vegetables
- Starchy vegetables
- Whole grains
- Nuts and seeds
- Peas, beans, lentils, and other legumes
- Fish, chicken, eggs, tofu, and other protein foods

- Avocados, olives, olive oil, and other heart-healthy fats

Of course, if you prefer to follow a special type of diet, such as a vegetarian, vegan, or pescatarian meal plan, you can adapt FMP menus to match your personalized needs and preferences.

Receive Custom Meal Plans

With the Fit Mother Project, you receive custom meal plans based on your lifestyle, health, and weight management goals.

As a rule, you will fill half of each plate with non-starchy vegetables, one-fourth of your plate with fiber-rich starches, and the remaining one-fourth of your plate with nutritious protein foods.

When losing weight using Fit Mother Project meal plans, you don't have to worry about nutritional deficiencies or fatigue.

In fact, your energy levels can drastically increase when choosing well-balanced weight loss plans.

Get Motivational Support

Staying motivated for weight loss is often half the battle, as your emotions can get in the way of achieving your ideal weight.

As a member of the Fit Mother Project, you receive newsletters and email motivational support from health experts, to increase your chance of staying on track with weight loss and healthy eating plans.

You also have access to private FMP social media groups, including motivational support from fit moms just like you.

If you suffer from chronic stress, anxiety, or depression that affects eating patterns and your calorie intake, see a doctor about possible mental health treatments that can relax you or boost your mood and motivation level during weight loss.

Gain Fat-Burning Workouts

Changing up your diet isn't the only necessary part of getting and staying healthy and lean.

Regular exercise is crucial for achieving your goal weight and maintaining it for life.

With the Fit Mother Project, you have access to a wide variety of fat-burning workouts specifically designed with busy women's needs in mind.

If you make time for at least 30 minutes of exercise daily, you can optimize the results of healthy eating changes.

Additionally, try to stay moving throughout the entire day — not just during workouts.

Aim to complete at least 45 minutes of daily activities that keep your body in motion, such as house chores, outdoor yard work, grocery shopping, cooking, or walking the dog.

Have Access to Healthy Recipes

Knowing how to prepare nutritious foods that taste delicious is important for long-term weight loss maintenance and chronic disease reduction.

With Fit Mother Project plans you receive healthy, well-balanced, delicious recipes your entire family will love!

FMP recipes are loaded with protein, fiber, healthy fats, vitamins, and minerals so you won't feel deprived or tired during your weight loss journey.

Take Dietary Supplements

The importance of taking dietary supplements during weight loss is two-fold.

Supplements can reduce your risk of vitamin, mineral, and other nutritional deficiencies and maximize energy levels.

Some weight loss supplements for women, such as protein bars, protein shakes, and fiber supplements, help boost satiety making it easier to eat fewer calories for weight loss.

Receive Health and Nutrition Education

Sometimes simply knowing more about nutrition and fitness, and how to ensure you ingest the right essential nutrients for your body, is one of the best ways to drop weight, stay healthy, and lower your risk of developing a chronic disease.

The Fit Mother Project offers nutrition education and email support from medical experts, and weekly newsletters to keep you up-to-date on ways to optimize the nutritional content of your diet, achieve your goal weight, and stay healthy for life.

Set Goals

Setting goals is one of the best ways to reach the bodyweight you desire.

Studies show that goal setting leads to greater long-term weight loss compared with not setting goals.

Choose goals for weekly weigh-ins, waist circumference, minutes of exercise completed, hours of sleep, and nutrition goals.

Aim to lose about 1-2 pounds weekly to drop weight at a safe, effective rate and achieve a goal weight you can maintain for life.

Set goals to avoid sugary drinks, sweets, highly processed foods, fried foods, refined grains, alcoholic drinks, and many fast foods.

You might allow yourself a cheat day every now and then but eliminate junk food as much as possible.

Self-Monitor

Self-monitor health and fitness parameters to keep track of weight loss progress throughout your journey.

Record your food intake, minutes exercised, hours of sleep, body weight, and more in a journal to keep yourself accountable for reaching the goals you set for yourself.

Studies show that daily weigh-ins are more effective for weight loss than weighing in less frequently.

Listen to Your Body

Whether you're following the Mayr Method diet or the Fit Mother Project eating plan, it's important to listen to your body when it comes to nutrition, fitness, sleep, and overall health and wellness.

If you feel hungry, eat a healthy snack or meal and stop eating when you feel full.

Your body might crave foods rich in vitamin C, such as citrus fruits, or protein-rich foods like chicken, fish, eggs, or tofu when it needs more of these essential nutrients.

Is the Mayr Method Diet Right for You?

While Rebel Wilson and other celebrities have touted success while following Mayr Method meal plans, the diet isn't for everybody.

If it's too restrictive for your taste, know you have additional, well-balanced options.

Many of the principals used in the Mayr Method plan, such as eating whole foods, reducing added sugar, getting regular exercise, and using mindfulness while eating, are components worth adopting regardless of your body weight and fitness goals.

Gut Health

Gut health is the cornerstone of our overall health. If your gut is out of whack, it can cause all sorts of problems, from eczema to autoimmune diseases.

Whether you're experiencing gut health issues yourself, or you just want more information, browse my gut health tips and information to help you understand how to heal your gut and start feeling better faster.

If you're reading this, you already know that gut health is the foundation for your overall health and wellness. But what's the best gut health diet?

What are the best gut healing foods? What should you be eating if you want to improve your gut health? What foods should you avoid for a healthy gut diet? You need answers so you can heal your gut, stay regular and achieve your best health.

What's the Best Gut Health Diet?

1. Change Your Diet – Heal Your Gut

2. The 4 F's of Gut Health

3. Fermented Foods

4. Fiber

5. Fruit

6. Foundation Foods

7. Quick List of the Best Foods for Gut Health

1. Change Your Diet – Heal Your Gut

What you eat determines which bacteria thrive in your gut. And research tells us that the good bacteria get stronger when we feed them the right foods.

Did you know that your body can create a new gut microbiota, in just 24 hours – by changing what you eat?

This means that even a lifetime of bad eating is fixable — at least as far as your gut microbes are concerned.

So, it's never too late to start healing your gut. Improving your gut health can help you feel better, lose weight, provide sustained energy and clear up a host of health maladies.

2. The 4 F's of Gut Health

So how can you keep your digestive system feeling good and functioning optimally? What are the best foods for gut health?

When it comes to foods that help promote a healthy gut, there are two main categories you'll want to focus on:

- **Probiotics:** These repopulate your gut with good bacteria.

- **Prebiotics:** These are food for your good gut bacteria. Prebiotics are fibers that we don't digest ourselves, so they are consumed by the good bacteria in our gut.

Taken together, prebiotic and probiotic foods work together to create a healthier, happier gut. If probiotics vs prebiotics seem confusing, it's worth the extra reading to figure it out!

The key foods are easy to remember if we break them down into four main groups.

I like to call them the 4 F's you need to heal your gut:

1. Fermented Foods

2. Fiber

3. Fruit

4. Foundation Foods

#1: Fermented Foods

Fermented foods are all the rage right now – and for good reason!

Fermentation not only creates a wide range of tangy, zingy, spicy foods, but it also results in a natural source of probiotics. These fermented foods provide natural probiotics or good gut bacteria to repopulate your healing gut.

#2: Fiber

Fiber – Fiber is a natural prebiotic which acts as the food for good bacteria. These fiber-based prebiotics are found in certain fruits, vegetables, and whole grains

#3: Fruits

While fruit is a healthy choice, there are a few fruits that are head and shoulders above the rest when it comes to gut health.

#4: Foundation Foods

These are nutrient-dense foods that are super healthy for your gut. Once you've fleshed out your diet with probiotic and prebiotic foods, these foundation foods give you the extra oomph you need to get your gut health back on track.

3. Fermented Foods

Fermented foods supply your digestive system with lots of healthy, living microorganisms to crowd out the accumulated unhealthy bacteria, and support overall health.

Fermentation is a process that's been around for centuries. Our ancestors discovered long ago, probably by accident, that fermenting foods was a great way to preserve them and make them last longer than just a season.

When foods ferment, they create lactic acid or alcohol, which helps to preserve the food. In the process, fermentation produces large amounts of probiotics, which are a bonus for your gut.

As a super added bonus, the fermentation process also adds additional nutrients to foods.

Fermented foods are trending for a reason. They inoculate your gut with healthy live bacteria and microorganisms that help heal your gut, crowd out the bad bacteria and give a boost to your overall health.

Here are some powerhouse fermented foods that you can easily add to your gut health diet to supercharge your gut health plan:

- **Sauerkraut:** Sauerkraut (or fermented cabbage) is a staple in German cuisine. You can find it in almost any grocery store, but it's even better to stick with freshly fermented varieties from health food stores to achieve the full nutrient value. It's easy to find recipes for homemade versions if you are crafty in the kitchen. As a nutrient bonus, sauerkraut is high in B vitamins and can help in the absorption of iron. Pile it on a hot dog, Reuben sandwich, or use it to season just about any grain, legume, scramble, meat, or vegetable dish.

- **Tempeh:** A fermented soy-based food that's been around for centuries, tempeh is becoming easier to find these days, with more and more restaurants creating with it and more stores stocking it on shelves. Tempeh is great in salads, on sandwiches, or as a tasty bacon alternative. Just make sure you thoroughly cook tempeh before you eat it. You may need to season it with a heavy hand because plain tempeh can be very bland.

- **Miso:** It may surprise you that this traditional Japanese soybean paste is a probiotic powerhouse. I had my first taste of miso in a soup at a Japanese restaurant. Beyond soup, this soybean paste has a whole host of uses in the kitchen. Miso paste can be used to make soup, added to salad dressings, or turned into a healthy mustard or plant-based miso-mayo. Whenever you choose soy-based products, remember to choose organic because most non-organic soy is genetically modified.

- **Kefir:** Kefir is a cultured, fermented beverage that tastes a lot like a thinner yogurt drink. It's made using starter grains, just as sourdough bread is made from a starter. Kefir is most commonly made with dairy milk, but it can be made with non-dairy alternatives including coconut milk, rice milk, coconut water, and goat's milk. Because it's a fermented product, even people who are lactose intolerant can tolerate dairy based kefir. Kefir is another product that you can DIY at home to make your own tasty probiotic. Just make sure you don't add much sugar to it or you'll be negating its good effect on your gut bacteria.

- **Pickles:** The humble pickle is another great probiotic food choice. Pickles, whether they are the cucumber variety, or made from other vegetables, are high in antioxidants, good gut bugs, and probiotics. But not all pickled foods are fermented. Stick with fresh varieties that are sold in the refrigerated section to make sure that the good bacteria are alive and that the nutrients stay intact. Try making your own pickles. My grandma was a champion pickle maker and she passed down all her recipes to me. Delicious and satisfying to make yourself.

- **Yogurt:** Yogurt is a naturally fermented food that can offer some serious probiotic power if you choose the right kinds. While most yogurts contain bacteria, make sure you look for a yogurt that has at least 1 billion live or active colony-forming units (CFUs) on the label. And stay away from the yogurts loaded with sugar, since sugar is bad for your healing gut.

- **Kimchi:** Kimchi is a spicy Korean alternative to sauerkraut. Kimchi is fermented cabbage made with several different spices like salt, chili powder, onion, garlic, and ginger. Studies have shown that this fermented cabbage Korean staple is rich in two strains of good bacteria associated with better gut health: Lactobacillus and Bifidobacterium. Kimchi adds a spicy kick to just about anything.

Tip: Many of these fermented foods are high in salt, so think about eating small portions of fermented foods daily and using them as a source of salt, replacing table salt, soy sauce, or other salt sources with pickled vegetables.

4. Fiber

Fiber is the most crucial ingredient for gut health. Unfortunately, only 3% of Americans get the recommended 40 grams of fiber they need each day.

Fiber is a potent pre-biotic, feeding the good bacteria your gut needs to be healthy.

Fiber is also a warrior in the battle against diverticulitis, the inflammation of the intestine. According to a medical study, eating insoluble fiber-rich foods has been found to reduce the risk of diverticulitis by an impressive 40%

Here are some of the best prebiotic powerhouses to add to your gut health diet:

- Beans: Beans feed good gut bacteria, which in turn revs up your immune system. They are packed with fiber, protein, folate, and B vitamins, which play a role in regulating a healthy gut and a healthy brain.

- **Polenta:** Polenta, or cornmeal mush is high in fiber and delicious. Polenta's insoluble fiber travels directly to the colon, where it ferments into multiple types of gut bacteria.

- **Flaxseed**: Flaxseed fuels your good gut flora, contains soluble fiber and can help improve digestive regularity. You've got to eat flaxseed ground up, or the seeds will pass through your digestive tract without being digested at all. Add ground flaxseed to smoothies or salads.

Keep your flaxseed in the refrigerator because once it's ground, it can go rancid fast.

- **Jicama:** This sweet, crunchy root vegetable is packed with fiber. One cup of raw jicama adds a whopping 6g of fiber to your diet. High in vitamin C, jicama is also great for weight loss and blood sugar control. Add it to salads, stir-fries or enjoy it as a crunchy snack.

• **Jerusalem artichokes:** Also known as sunroot, sunchoke, or earth apple, the Jerusalem artichoke is high in inulin, an insoluble fiber. Inulin travels to the colon where it ferments into healthy good bacteria. You can cook Jerusalem artichokes like a potato or shred it raw and add it to salads. Beware though: Start small with this vegetable because it can cause gas until your gut adjusts

5. Fruit

Most fruits are healthy options, but these three are powerful additions to your gut health diet.

• Apples: Not only are apples available nearly everywhere, but they are also an excellent addition to a gut health diet.

They are high in fiber, and a recent study found green apples boost good gut bacteria.

Stewed apples have been found to be good for your microbiome, and they may also help to heal your gut. An apple a day really can keep the doctor away.

- **Blueberries:** Blueberries are little delicious bombs of healthy goodness. A well-known superfood, blueberries are full of antioxidants, vitamin K compounds, and fiber. If that weren't enough, studies have shown that blueberries also diversify our gut bacteria.

- **Bananas:** Bananas have long been a standard prescription for an upset stomach. That's because compounds in bananas work to maintain harmony in your gut microbiome. Bananas may also reduce inflammation, due to high levels of potassium and magnesium.

So, slice some on your oatmeal, throw one in a smoothie, or keep them on hand for a midday snack.

6. Foundation Foods

Now that you've got your Fermented, Fiber and Fruit foods in line, here are other good choices to add to your gut health diet. All of these foods are great foundation foods because they are nutrient dense foods that also support your gut healing diet.

- Broccoli
- Dandelion Greens
- Asparagus
- Seaweed
- Garlic, onions, scallions
- Gum Arabic
- Barley
- Shirataki Noodles
- Cacao
- Wheat Bran
- Chicory Root
- Chickpeas
- Oatmeal

7. Summary of the Best Foods for Gut Health

Start adding these foods to your daily gut health routine and you'll be on your way to a happy, healthy gut in no time.

Fermented Foods or Probiotics

- Sauerkraut
- Tempeh
- Miso
- Pickles
- Kefir
- Yogurt
- Kimchi

Fiber-rich Foods or Prebiotics

- Beans
- Polenta
- Flaxseed
- Jicama
- Jerusalem Artichokes

Fruits

- Apples
- Blueberries
- Bananas

Foundation Foods or Nutrient Dense Foods

- Broccoli
- Dandelion Greens
- Asparagus
- Seaweed
- Garlic, onions, scallions
- Gum Arabic
- Barley
- Shirataki Noodles
- Cacao
- Wheat Bran
- Chicory Root
- Chickpeas
- Oatmeal

CHAPTER THREE

Intermittent Fasting

What is intermittent fasting and does it actually work?

Intermittent fasting is one of the best ways I've found to lose weight and not feel like I'm on a crazy diet. Intermittent fasting benefits are backed by scientific research and the results from intermittent fasting are pretty amazing.

If you are looking for more information on the different types of intermittent fasting, the pros and cons of intermittent fasting, what to eat while fasting, and things to watch out for if you are a woman who wants to try intermittent fasting, you've come to the right place.

What is intermittent fasting?

Intermittent fasting involves cycling between periods of eating and fasting.

Most types of this dietary pattern focus on limiting your meals and snacks to a specific time window — typically between 6 and 8 hours of the day.

For example, 16/8 intermittent fasting involves restricting food intake to just 8 hours per day and abstaining from eating during the remaining 16 hours.

Other types involve fasting for 24 hours once or twice per week or significantly cutting calorie intake a few days per week but eating normally during the others.

Although most people practice intermittent fasting to enhance weight loss, it has been associated with many other health benefits as well. In fact, studies show that intermittent fasting may improve blood sugar levels, decrease cholesterol, and boost longevity.

Note: Intermittent fasting is a popular eating pattern that restricts your food intake to a specific time window. It doesn't limit the types or amount of food you eat.

Does it work for weight loss?

Several studies show that intermittent fasting may boost weight loss via several mechanisms.

First, restricting your meals and snacks to a strict time window may naturally decrease your calorie intake, which can aid weight loss.

Intermittent fasting may also increase levels of norepinephrine, a hormone and neurotransmitter that can boost your metabolism to increase calorie burning throughout the day.

Furthermore, this eating pattern may reduce levels of insulin, a hormone involved in blood sugar management. Decreased levels can bump up fat burning to promote weight loss.

Some research even shows that intermittent fasting can help your body retain muscle mass more effectively than calorie restriction, which may increase its appeal.

According to one review, intermittent fasting may reduce body weight by up to 8% and decrease body fat by up to 16% over 3-12 weeks.

Synergy with keto

When paired with the ketogenic diet, intermittent fasting can speed up ketosis and amplify weight loss.

The keto diet, which is very high in fats but low in carbs, is designed to kick-start ketosis.

Ketosis is a metabolic state that forces your body to burn fat for fuel instead of carbs. This occurs when your body is deprived of glucose, which is its main source of energy.

Combining intermittent fasting with the keto diet can help your body enter ketosis faster to maximize results. It can likewise mitigate some of the side effects that often occur when starting this diet, including the keto flu, which is characterized by nausea, headaches, and fatigue.

Note: Research indicates that intermittent fasting can increase weight loss by boosting fat burning and metabolism. When used in tandem with the ketogenic diet, it may help speed up ketosis to maximize weight loss.

Other benefits

Intermittent fasting has also been linked to several other health benefits. It may:

• **Improve heart health.** Intermittent fasting has been shown to decrease levels of total and LDL (bad) cholesterol, as well as triglycerides, all of which are risk factors for heart disease.

• **Support blood sugar control.** A small study in 10 people with type 2 diabetes noted that intermittent fasting helped significantly decrease blood sugar levels.

• **Decrease inflammation.** Several studies have found that this eating pattern may reduce specific blood markers of inflammation.

• **Increase longevity.** Although research in humans is lacking, some animal studies suggest that intermittent fasting may boost your lifespan and slow signs of aging.

- **Protect brain function.** Studies in mice reveal that this dietary pattern may improve brain function and combat conditions like Alzheimer's disease.

- **Increase human growth hormone.** Intermittent fasting may naturally increase levels of human growth hormone (HGH), which can help improve body composition and metabolism

Note: Intermittent fasting is associated with numerous health benefits, including decreased inflammation, increased heart and brain health, and better blood sugar control.

Potential downsides

Most people can practice intermittent fasting safely as part of a healthy lifestyle. However, it may not be the best choice for everyone.

Children, individuals with a chronic illness, and women who are pregnant or breastfeeding should consult a healthcare professional before starting this dietary pattern to ensure that they're getting the nutrients they need.

People with diabetes should also exercise caution, as fasting can lead to dangerous drops in blood sugar levels and may interfere with certain medications.

While athletes and those who are physically active can safely practice intermittent fasting, it's best to plan meals and fast days around intense workouts to optimize physical performance.

Finally, this lifestyle pattern may not be as effective for women. In fact, human and animal studies indicate that intermittent fasting may negatively affect women's blood sugar control, contribute to menstrual-cycle abnormalities, and decrease fertility.

Note: Although intermittent fasting is generally safe and effective, it may not be right for everyone. Notably, some studies suggest that it could have several adverse effects in women.

How Intermittent Fasting Can Help You Lose Weight

There are many different ways to lose weight.

One strategy that has become popular in recent years is called intermittent fasting.

Intermittent fasting is an eating pattern that involves regular, short-term fasts — or periods of minimal or no food consumption.

Most people understand intermittent fasting as a weight loss intervention. Fasting for short periods of time helps people eat fewer calories, which may result in weight loss over time.

However, intermittent fasting may also help modify risk factors for health conditions like diabetes and cardiovascular disease, such as lowering cholesterol and blood sugar levels

Choosing your intermittent fasting plan

There are several different intermittent fasting methods. The most popular ones include:

- The 16:8 method

- The 5:2 diet
- The Warrior diets
- Eat Stop Eat
- Alternate-day fasting (ADF)

All methods can be effective, but figuring out which one works best depends on the individual.

To help you choose the method that fits your lifestyle, here's a breakdown of the pros and cons of each.

The 16/8 method

The 16/8 intermittent fasting plan is one of the most popular styles of fasting for weight loss.

The plan restricts food consumption and calorie-containing beverages to a set window of 8 hours per day. It requires abstaining from food for the remaining 16 hours of the day.

While other diets can set strict rules and regulations, the 16/8 method is based on a time-restricted feeding (TRF) model and more flexible.

You can choose any 8-hour window to consume calories.

Some people opt to skip breakfast and fast from noon to 8 p.m., while others avoid eating late and stick to a 9 a.m. to 5 p.m. schedule.

Limiting the number of hours that you can eat during the day may help you lose weight and lower your blood pressure.

Research indicates that time-restricted feeding patterns such as the 16/8 method may prevent hypertension and reduce the amount of food consumed, leading to weight loss.

A 2016 study found that when combined with resistance training, the 16/8 method helped decreased fat mass and maintain muscle mass in male participants.

A more recent study found that the 16/8 method did not impair gains in muscle or strength in women performing resistance training.

While the 16/8 method can easily fit into any lifestyle, some people may find it challenging to avoid eating for 16 hours straight.

Additionally, eating too many snacks or junk food during your 8-hour window can negate the positive effects associated with 16/8 intermittent fasting.

Be sure to eat a balanced diet comprising fruits, vegetables, whole grains, healthy fats, and protein to maximize the potential health benefits of this diet.

The 5:2 method

The 5:2 diet is a straightforward intermittent fasting plan.

Five days per week, you eat normally and don't restrict calories. Then, on the other two days of the week, you reduce your calorie intake to one-quarter of your daily needs.

For someone who regularly consumes 2,000 calories per day, this would mean reducing their calorie intake to just 500 calories per day, two days per week.

According to a 2018 study, the 5:2 diet is just as effective as daily calorie restriction for weight loss and blood glucose control among those with type 2 diabetes.

Another study found that the 5:2 diet was just as effective as continuous calorie restriction for both weight loss and the prevention of metabolic diseases like heart disease and diabetes.

The 5:2 diet provides flexibility, as you get to pick which days you fast, and there are no rules regarding what or when to eat on full-calorie days.

That said, it's worth mentioning that eating "normally" on full-calorie days does not give you a free pass to eat whatever you want.

Restricting yourself to just 500 calories per day isn't easy, even if it's only for two days per week. Plus, consuming too few calories may make you feel ill or faint.

The 5:2 diet can be effective, but it's not for everyone. Talk to your doctor to see if the 5:2 diet may be right for you.

Eat Stop Eat

Eat Stop Eat is an unconventional approach to intermittent fasting popularized by Brad Pilon, author of the book "Eat Stop Eat."

This intermittent fasting plan involves identifying one or two non-consecutive days per week during which you abstain from eating, or fast, for a 24-hour period.

During the remaining days of the week, you can eat freely, but it's recommended to eat a well-rounded diet and avoid overconsumption.

The rationale behind a weekly 24-hour fast is that consuming fewer calories will lead to weight loss.

Fasting for up to 24 hours can lead to a metabolic shift that causes your body to use fat as an energy source instead of glucose.

But avoiding food for 24 hours at a time requires a lot of willpower and may lead to binging and overconsumption later on. It may also lead to disordered eating patterns.

More research is needed regarding the Eat Stop Eat diet to determine its potential health benefits and weight loss properties.

Talk to your doctor before trying Eat Stop Eat to see if it may be an effective weight loss solution for you.

Alternate-day fasting

Alternate-day fasting is an intermittent fasting plan with an easy-to-remember structure. On this diet, you fast every other day but can eat whatever you want on the non-fasting days.

Some versions of this diet embrace a "modified" fasting strategy that involves eating around 500 calories on fasting days. However, other versions eliminate calories altogether on fasting days.

Alternate-day fasting has proven weight loss benefits.

A randomized pilot study comparing alternate-day fasting to a daily caloric restriction in adults with obesity found both methods to be equally effective for weight loss.

Another study found that participants consumed 35% fewer calories and lost an average of 7.7 pounds (3.5 kg) after alternating between 36 hours of fasting and 12 hours of unlimited eating over 4 weeks.

If you really want to maximize weight loss, adding an exercise regime to your life can help.

Research shows that combining alternate-day fasting with endurance exercise may cause twice as much weight loss than simply fast.

A full fast every other day can be extreme, especially if you're new to fasting. Overeating on non-fasting days can also be tempting.

If you're new to intermittent fasting, ease into alternate-day fasting with a modified fasting plan.

Whether you start with a modified fasting plan or full fast, it's best to maintain a nutritious diet, incorporating high protein foods and low-calorie vegetables to help you feel full.

The Warrior diets

The Warrior Diet is an intermittent fasting plan based on the eating patterns of ancient warriors.

Created in 2001 by Ori Hofmekler, the Warrior Diet is a bit more extreme than the 16:8 method but less restrictive than the Eat Fast Eat method.

It consists of eating very little for 20 hours during the day, and then eating as much food as desired throughout a 4-hour window at night.

The Warrior Diet encourages dieters to consume small amounts of dairy products, hard-boiled eggs, and raw fruits and vegetables, as well as non-calorie fluids during the 20-hour fast period.

After this 20-hour fast, people can essentially eat anything they want for a 4-hour window, but unprocessed, healthy, and organic foods are recommended.

While there's no research on the Warrior Diet specifically, human studies indicate that time-restricted feeding cycles can lead to weight loss.

Time-restricted feeding cycles may have a variety of other health benefits. Studies show that time-restricted feeding cycles can prevent diabetes, slow tumor progression, delay aging, and increase lifespan in rodents.

More research is needed on the Warrior Diet to fully understand its benefits for weight loss.

The Warrior Diet may be difficult to follow, as it restricts substantial calorie consumption to just 4 hours per day. Overconsumption at night is a common challenge.

The Warrior Diet may also lead to disordered eating patterns. If you feel up for the challenge, talk to your doctor to see whether it's right for you.

The Takeaway: Is the Mayr Method Healthy?

Continuously converse with your doctor before you make any change to your diet or wellbeing plan.

Since the Mayr program focuses on methods that are proven to improve your overall health like intermittent fasting, improving your gut health, and expanding your mindfulness and focus at supper time, it shouldn't be harmful. Again, always speak to your health professional before you start any health program.

I've never tried the Mayr technique, yet aside from counting my biting, I don't think it would be too far outside my wheelhouse since I as of now love irregular fasting and gut health topics.

On the off chance that I had an extra couple thousand dollars lying around, I wouldn't disdain checking into an extravagance Austrian spa for a few days to check out the program in person.

I'd love to hear your take on the program on the off chance that you've attempted it. On the off chance that you'd like to improve your health without jumping on the Mayr bandwagon, check out these resource libraries for more information on gut health and intermittent fasting:

- Gut Health Resource Library
- Intermittent Fasting Resource Library

CONCLUSION

Irregular fasting has been shown to support digestion and fat burning while protecting slender body mass, all of which can help weight loss.

When joined with other slims down like the keto diet, it may additionally accelerate ketosis and reduce negative side effects, such as the keto influenza.

Although it may not work for everyone, intermittent fasting can be a safe and effective weight loss strategy.

Made in the USA
Middletown, DE
06 May 2022